Being Healthy, Feeling Great

# Exercise

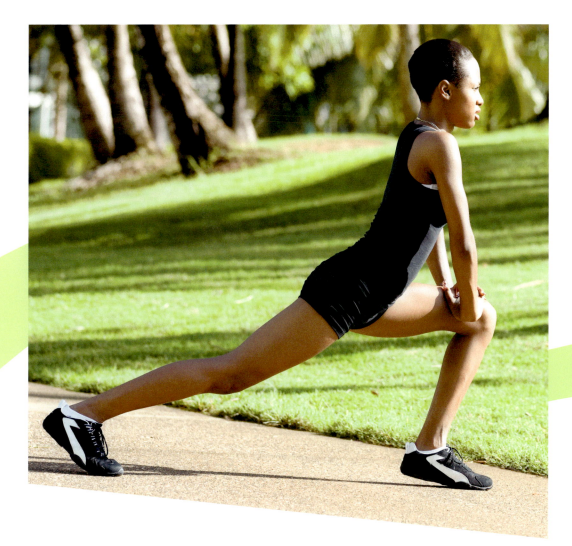

**Robyn Hardyman**

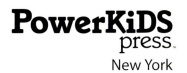
press™

New York

Published in 2010 by The Rosen Publishing Group Inc.
29 East 21st Street, New York, NY 10010

First Edition

Design: Nick Leggett and Paul Myerscough
Editor: Sarah Eason
Picture research: Maria Joannou
Illustrator: Geoff Ward
Consultant: Sue Beck, MSc, BSc
Commissioning Editor for Wayland: Jennifer Sanderson

Library of Congress Cataloging-in-Publication Data

Hardyman, Robyn.
Exercise / Robyn Hardyman.
p. cm. -- (Being healthy, feeling great)
Includes index.
ISBN 978-1-61532-368-5 (library binding)
ISBN 978-1-61532-374-6 (paperback)
ISBN 978-1-61532-375-3 (6-pack)
1. Exercise. I. Title.
GV481.H2553 2010
613.7'1--dc22

2009023889

Photographs:
The publisher would like to thank the following for permission to reproduce photographs:
Corbis: Charles Gullung/Zefa 14, Ariel Skelley 7; Fotolia: Galina Barskaya 24; Istockphoto: Ana
Abejon 18, Chris Schmidt 11, Jacom Stephens 1, 17, Bob Thomas 4, 31; Rex Features: Image Source
12; Shutterstock: Galina Barskaya 19, Archana Bhartia 26, Jacek Chabraszewski 16, Cathleen
Clapper 5, Stephen Coburn 23, Mandy Godbehear 20, Marilyn Barbone 8, Monkey Business Images
13, Juriah Mosin 10, 17, Amy Myers 27, Photocreo/Michal Bednarek 25, Lee Prince 21, Dragan
Trifunovic 6, Peter Weber 9, 22. Cover: Shutterstock/Gert Johannes Jacobus Vrey

Manufactured in China

CPSIA Compliance Information: Batch #WAW0102PK: For Further Information

contact Rosen Publishing, New York, New York at 1-800-237-9932

# Contents

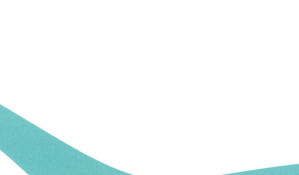

# Exercise for life!

Exercise is any kind of physical activity you do that makes your body strong and healthy. Exercise is really important, because it keeps you fit. When your body is fit, it helps you to fight sickness, so you stay well, too. On top of all this, exercise can be really fun!

## Healthy habits!

Exercise is one of the healthiest habits you can have. It makes you feel great! In fact, the more you exercise, the more you want to exercise. This is because exercise makes your body feel at its best. You feel fit and healthy. You find it easier to do all the things you have to do in a day, from tying your shoelaces to going to school.

Exercise as part of a team can be a lot of fun and helps to keep you motivated, too.

## Live longer

People who exercise as part of their routine often take care of themselves in other ways, too. They often eat a healthy diet, because they know this is good for them. Adults who do regular exercise and eat healthily are less likely to develop serious illnesses, such as heart disease, as they get older. They are more likely to live longer than adults who do not have the same healthy habits.

## Couch potato?

People who spend too much of their time just sitting still, watching lots of television or playing computer games, are sometimes called "couch potatoes." Because they do not do much—or any—exercise, they become unfit. Their bodies become weaker and they may put on weight.

## Amazing fact

An active adult takes at least 10,000 steps a day! An active child will probably take 13,000 to 15,000 steps each day. You can measure how far you have walked or many steps you take in a day by using a small device called a pedometer.

Exercising is a good habit to get into. It is easier if the whole family joins in!

# What is exercise?

You may think that exercise is all about sports and that it has to be hard work. But exercise is any kind of activity you do that makes your body work a little harder than usual. If you feel slightly out of breath and a little bit warm, and if your heart is beating a little faster when you are still, you are exercising.

## The right level

There are three different levels of exercise. Some types of exercise, such as walking at normal speed, are gentle. Cycling and dancing are moderate types of exercise. Doing vigorous exercise, such as running and swimming fast, makes your body work hardest.

Any exercise is good for you. If you are not used to doing much exercise, start with gentle activities and move on to more vigorous exercise later.

Dance classes or just dancing to music is good exercise.

## Lots of choice

You can choose between all kinds of exercise, from playing sports, such as tennis and football, to jump rope. You could walk to school, too. Remember, anything that makes your body work harder is exercise.

You can exercise alone or with other people. Dancing to your favorite music in your bedroom is a fun way to exercise on your own. Kicking a ball around with friends in the park or swimming together are ways to enjoy exercise with friends. Families can exercise together, too—by going for a walk or a bicycle ride.

## Anyone can do it

Exercise is for everyone! People of all ages and abilities and all shapes and sizes can have fun and get fit by being more active.

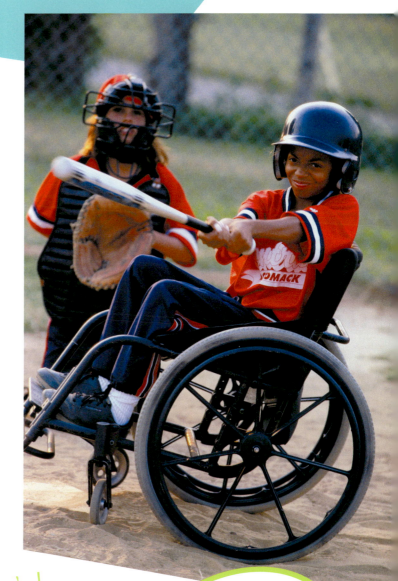

Able-bodied people and disabled people alike should all do regular exercise.

**Healthy Hints**

### Doing enough?

Keep a record of how much exercise you take every day for a week. Are you doing enough? School-age children should aim to do moderate or vigorous exercise for one hour each day.

# Exercise for health

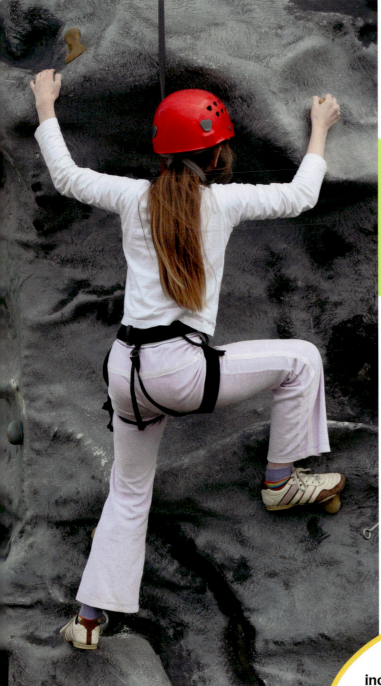

Different types of exercise improve strength, stamina, and flexibility. You need all three to be truly fit, which is why you need to try a variety of exercises.

## Getting stronger

Exercise makes your body's muscles stronger. This makes it easier for you to lift or carry things, such as your school bag. Strong muscles can also protect your joints. This means you are much less likely to hurt yourself when you run or bend over quickly.

Different types of exercise use different muscles. For example, cycling uses your leg muscles most. Swimming is great exercise because it uses many different muscles in your legs, arms, and the rest of your body. Some adults lift weights to increase muscle strength, but this is not a suitable exercise for young people.

Rock climbing increases your muscle strength and improves your flexibility.

## Keep going for longer

Exercise improves your stamina. Stamina is your ability to keep doing a physical activity for a long time. When you exercise, your heart and lungs have to work harder. This makes them stronger and more effective. More blood and oxygen can be pumped around your body to all your other muscles. This gives them the energy they need to move.

When you first start to exercise, you may get out of breath and feel tired quickly. As you exercise more, you will find that you can keep going for longer. This is because you have more stamina—you are getting fitter! Swimming, football, and basketball are examples of exercise that builds stamina.

## Twist and bend

Exercise makes your body more flexible. This means that it can bend and stretch easily. If you do not move your body much, your tendons become tight. It is much harder to do simple things, such as putting on socks. Yoga, ballet, and martial arts are all good forms exercise that improve flexibility.

**Long-distance running is an excellent way to increase your stamina.**

## Amazing fact

When you do exercise, your heart pumps blood around your body twice as quickly as when you are resting.

# Exercise for fun

The key to exercising regularly is finding an exercise that you like. You are much more likely to continue exercising if you choose something you find fun and enjoyable.

## Take your pick

Everyone is different. Not everyone likes baseball, gymnastics, or tennis. Some people dislike team sports. Others do not like exercising on their own. Fortunately, there are many types of exercise to choose from.

Take a look at the types of exercise in the box below. Can you find some forms of exercise you enjoy and that improve your strength, stamina, and flexibility?

| Exercise | Stamina | Strength | Flexibility |
|---|---|---|---|
| Walking | ● | ● | |
| Cycling | ● | ● | |
| Swimming | ● | ● | ● |
| Dancing | ● | | ● |
| Football | ● | | |
| Basketball | ● | ● | ● |
| Running | ● | ● | |
| Tennis | ● | ● | ● |
| Yoga | | ● | ● |

Simple playground fun can make your body stronger and fitter.

## Going solo

If you prefer to exercise on your own, there are plenty of forms of exercise to choose from. Good options include running, cycling, and swimming.

## With other people

If you prefer exercising in a group, why not try team sports such as basketball, football, baseball, soccer, and hockey? You should be able to find a team to join in your school or local community.

If you want to get fit with a friend, why not try tennis, badminton, or table tennis? You could run or swim with a friend, too—sometimes having someone else to exercise with can help you to keep it up.

### Jump rope

**Healthy Hints**

Jump roping is a fun way to keep fit—and all you need is a piece of rope!

Winning a sport event is great motivation—you will want to train even harder to win again!

# Exercise to feel good

Exercise helps your body to become strong and healthy. Being active has other benefits, too, which can make you feel really good in different ways.

## A sense of achievement

When you first start exercising, it can feel a little like hard work. Your muscles, lungs, and heart are not used to the extra effort and they become tired quickly. As you keep exercising, you soon find that it becomes easier. You will become stronger and fitter. And as you get fitter, you will start to feel more confident. You may also feel proud because you know that you have achieved something really good.

Like everything else you do, exercise takes practice. You have to learn skills involved in the sport or activity you are doing. When someone first gets on a skateboard, they may fall off. As they practice more, they learn to skateboard easily, and in time, they can learn great moves. This, too, is something to be proud of. It is good to see how much better you can get!

Exercise can seem hard, but it also feels good to push yourself.

## Stress-free zone

Exercise helps to reduce stress. This is because when you exercise, your brain releases special chemicals. They are called endorphins and they make you feel happy. When you are active, it makes it easier for you to relax and forget about anything that might be worrying you.

If you have had plenty of exercise during the day, you will usually sleep really well at night. When you have slept well, you will be better prepared for the day ahead. You will find it easier to concentrate on things you have to do, such as schoolwork.

**Need a boost?**

**Healthy Hints**

When you feel fed up, try doing some exercise —it will soon cheer you up!

If your body is fit and healthy, your brain is more likely to be fit, too.

# Before you start

No matter what kind of exercise you choose to do, it is important to prepare your body carefully before you start. If you rush straight into energetic exercise, it can damage your body. Doing warm-up exercises can help you to avoid injury.

## Warm up your body

The first part of any exercise is warming up your body. Any activity that makes you feel that you are sweating very slightly is a good way to start. Your body will definitely feel warmer by then, and your heart and lungs will be working a little harder. Try jogging in place for two minutes. Or spend a few minutes walking quickly, cycling, or dancing slowly.

Warm up with gentle exercise before you start any vigorous activity.

### Stretch...

**Healthy Hints**

To stretch your calves, stand a couple of steps away from a wall. Keep your heels flat on the ground, then lean against the wall with your hands touching it. Count to ten, and then rest. Repeat the stretch once or twice.

## Get stretching

When muscles are cold, they are not very stretchy. If you stretch cold muscles too far during exercise, you can strain them. So, the second part of warm-up exercises is spending a few minutes stretching your muscles. Do this only when you have already warmed up.

Touching your toes is a good way to stretch your muscles. You can do this a few times. Remember: do not overstretch—your muscle may feel like it is going to snap if you have gone too far. Do not hold your breath as you stretch.

## Practice your skills

The last part of warming up is spending a few minutes practicing some of the skills you will need when you do your main activity. For instance, you could try throwing, catching, or kicking a ball if you are playing a ball game.

## Cool down

Cool-down exercises help to protect your body, too. Before you stop exercising, spend a few minutes doing some stretching.

**Healthy Hints**

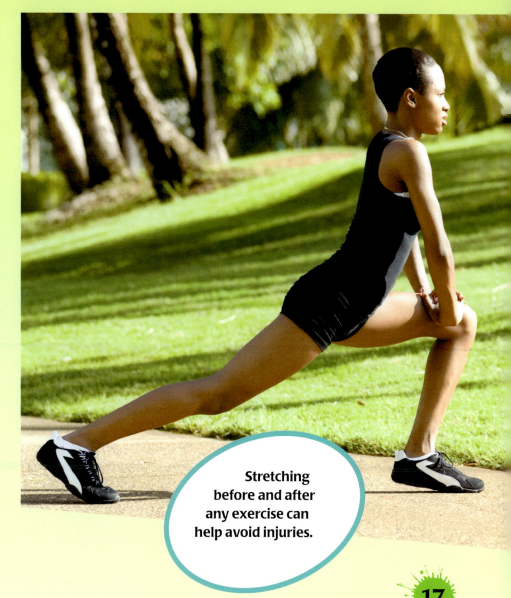

Stretching before and after any exercise can help avoid injuries.

17

# Exercises for stamina

Different kinds of exercise make you fit in different ways. Aerobic exercises make your heart beat faster. They make you breathe faster, too, so your lungs also have to work harder. Aerobic exercises help to build up your stamina so you can keep going for longer.

## Aerobic fun

There are lots of fun aerobic exercises to choose from. You could try walking quickly, jogging or running in a park or in the countryside with the rest of your family.

Cycling and roller-skating are other great ways to get your heart and lungs working well. Swimming is excellent aerobic exercise, too. Swimming does not make your joints work too hard, but it still gives you a really good aerobic workout. Some schools offer swimming lessons, or maybe you could go to swim at a pool near to where you live.

You use lots of muscles to swim, but you do not put pressure on joints.

Many team sports are forms of aerobic exercise. Try joining a volleyball or basketball team at school. Or join a hockey or rowing team in your local community. When you are part of a team, it helps you to keep going with exercise, even on days when you do not feel like exercising very much.

## Keep going

When you first start to do aerobic exercises, you may feel out of breath and tired really quickly. You may be able to run for just two or three minutes before you need to stop for a break. However, as you continue to exercise, your heart and lungs become more and more efficient. In time, you will also find that you can keep going for longer and longer.

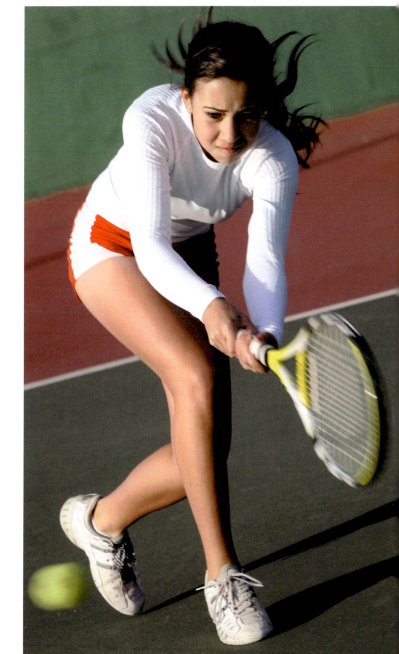

Tennis is an excellent aerobic exercise.

## Amazing fact

When you exercise, your lungs can take in more than ten times more air with each breath than they can when you are relaxed.

# Exercises for strength and flexibility

Aerobic exercises are good for helping you to get fit by improving your stamina. Other types of exercise work on your strength and flexibility. It is great to do a variety of different kinds of exercise, so that you work on all three elements of fitness. That way, you will give yourself the best chance you can to be healthy.

## Stronger muscles

Using your muscles makes them stronger. Strong muscles help your body to move more quickly. Strong muscles help you to lift and push things.

Climbing on a jungle gym and swinging on monkey bars in a park are really good ways to build up your strength. You could also do simple exercises at home, such as sit-ups and pushups. Running, jumping, and cycling also make your muscles much stronger and these exercises work your heart and lungs, too.

Strong muscles are needed to perform exercises such as handstands.

## Flexibility

When your body is flexible, it makes it easier for you to stretch and bend. This helps with all kinds of everyday activities, such as washing your back in the shower or in the bathtub.

You can increase your flexibility just by stretching more than usual. For example, if you have to stretch to get a book that is just out of reach, this makes your arms and back more flexible. You can do specific stretching exercises to help even more. Try doing side stretches or touching your toes.

Some sports are great for flexibility, too. Have you ever seen a gymnast do a backflip? They make it look easy! This is because gymnastics makes your body much more flexible. Martial arts are also a good choice. You can choose from many different types, such as judo and kung fu.

## A good variety

### Healthy Hints

Different exercises help to keep you fit in different ways. Running helps to keep your heart healthy, and stretching helps to keep you flexible. Trying different types keeps exercise fun.

Ballet is a great way to increase your flexibility.

# Getting warmer!

Exercise makes your body hotter. When your muscles work hard, they give off heat, and this heat spreads through your body. You can get too hot when exercising. Fortunately, your body has some clever ways of stopping you from overheating.

## Blood vessels

When you get hot, the small blood vessels near the surface of your skin get wider, so that more blood can flow through them. You may have noticed that you look flushed during exercise. This change in the blood vessels is the reason why. As the blood flows close to the skin's surface, it cools down. This helps your whole body to cool down a little, too.

## Sweating

If you exercise hard, you sweat. This is another way that your body helps to cool you down. Sweat passes from the inside to the outside of your body through pores, or tiny holes, in your skin. When sweat reaches the surface of your skin, it evaporates in the air. This cools your skin—and you do not feel as hot.

You get flushed and sweaty when you do vigorous exercise.

## Amazing fact

When you exercise, sweat is released through about 2.5 million pores in your skin!

## Help yourself!

If you begin to get overheated during exercise, it can make you feel unwell. You may feel nauseous, dizzy, and tired. You can avoid this by taking some simple measures.

When you sweat, you lose important liquid from your body. You can replace this by drinking water before, during, and after exercise. Remember, the more you sweat, the more you need to drink. On a hot day, it is helpful to exercise in the cooler parts of the day— in the morning or evening, for instance. If you keep a water bottle with you, you can also throw some water over your head to cool down.

**Keep a water bottle close at hand when you exercise.**

23

# The right amount

Exercise is good for you, because it helps you to get fit and stay healthy and it is a lot of fun, too! However, too much exercise can be harmful for your body. It is important to know how much exercise to do—and when to stop.

## Damaging muscles and joints

If you exercise too much, you may damage your muscles and joints. Stretching a joint too far may pull one of the muscles connected to it. A pulled muscle hurts when you move it. You should always stop if you feel any pain while exercising. If you pull a muscle, you should rest it until it is better. If your muscle still hurts after resting, see a doctor.

## Warning signs

There are other signs to look out for, too. If you feel dizzy or faint, stop exercising. Rest and drink plenty of water. Your body may be getting too hot. If you are really out of breath, or if you feel nauseous, you should also rest for a while.

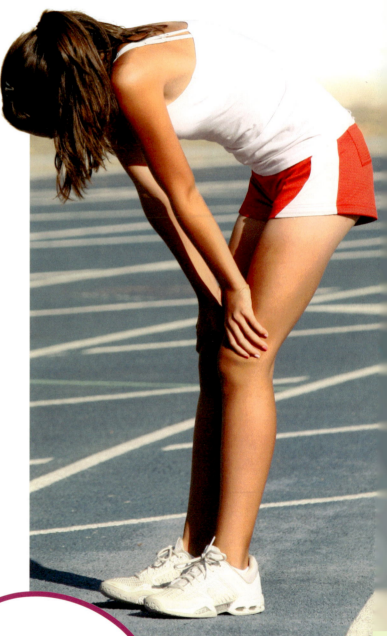

Vigorous exercise can make your body tired. Give it time to recover!

## When you are unwell

It is normal to feel unwell at times. If you feel unwell, it is best to avoid exercise until you feel better. Your body needs to work at recovering from the sickness, so let it do its job for a few days.

## Sleep and exercise

Top sports people know that getting enough sleep is very important in helping them to perform well. Sleep is essential for everybody. While you are still growing, you need a lot of sleep. Try to get at least ten or 11 hours' sleep a night. That way, your body will be rested and ready to exercise.

## Cramps

**Healthy Hints**

A cramp is when a muscle gets really tight and does not relax again. This can happen during exercise, and it can be very painful! Rubbing the area can help. Drinking plenty of water can help to stop cramps from happening.

Sleep is important—it is then that your body repairs itself.

# Exercising safely

When you exercise, make sure that you do it safely. By exercising safely, you will help to prevent any injury.

## Clothing and equipment

For some forms of exercise, you need the right clothing and equipment. For instance, you will need a swimsuit and towel to swim, and perhaps some goggles. To play football, you will need a football and helmet. For vigorous exercise, wear loose clothing made from material such as cotton. Wear suitable gym shoes, or the correct shoes for sports such as football or hockey.

For some activities, you need to wear protective equipment. For example, for skateboarding you need a helmet and knee and elbow pads.

If you are cycling, you will need a helmet. Try to wear reflective clothing, too, especially if you are cycling in the dark. Check your bicycle before you use it to make sure it is working properly.

**A cycling helmet will protect you if you have an accident.**

## Outdoors

If you exercise outdoors on a sunny day, be sure to put on sunscreen and a hat to protect yourself from the strong sun. Remember to drink plenty of water, too.

Always take lots of care when crossing streets. Stop, look, and listen before you cross. If you are cycling, be aware of other road users and follow the rules of the road. Whenever you go out to exercise, tell an adult where you are going and when you will be home.

## Follow the rules

Many kinds of exercise and sport have rules. These are for everyone's safety. Be sure to follow the rules at all times, and always listen to whoever is in charge. This will help to avoid accidents and injuries. When you exercise, think about other people. Do not do anything that could hurt anyone around you!

**Always exercise with friends, if you can—there is safety in numbers!**

## Remove jewelry

Jewelry, such as earrings, can get in the way during exercise. It is best to remove these items before you start.

**Healthy Hints**

# Warm-up exercises

Here are some examples of warm-up exercises. Remember to do some of them before you start your exercise.

**1** Bend your right knee and gently stretch out your left leg behind you, keeping your left foot on the ground. Lean on a wall with your hands, or rest them on your right thigh. Hold this stretch for 20 seconds. Switch over and do the same with the other leg.

**2** Place your left leg in front of you. Lift up your left foot, keeping your heel on the ground. With your right hand, hold onto the toes of your left foot for 20 seconds. Repeat on your right leg.

**3** Circle your arms around and around at the shoulders.

**4** Put your hands on your hips and twist your body at the waist. Twist five times in one direction, then five times in the other direction.

**5** Put your hands on your waist and gently bend over sideways, first to the right and then to the left. Do this five times on each side.

**6** Clasp your hands together and raise them directly above your head. Push upward gently to stretch your arms and shoulders.

**7** Stand on your right leg and bend your left leg behind you. Hold onto your left foot for 20 seconds. Repeat on the other leg.

**8** Hold your left arm across your body. Place your right arm under your left arm and pull your left arm toward your body. Repeat on the right arm.

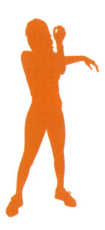

# Quiz

How much exercise do you do? Try this quick quiz to find out.

**1  It is recess at school. Do you:**

a) Stand around in the playground, on your own or with friends, until it is time to go back inside?
b) Walk around the playground with your best friend, talking about last night's television shows?
c) Get together with some friends and kick a ball around for as long as you can?

**2  You get home from school and it is raining outside. Do you:**

a) Switch on the television and watch for an hour or two—preferably, with a bag of candy?
b) Play on the computer for a while, then dance to your favorite music in your room?
c) Ask your parent to take you to the pool to swim?

**3  You have an important test at school tomorrow. Do you:**

a) Stay up studying until late, then lie awake worrying about it?
b) Do some studying when you get home, then go to bed early?
c) Play an energetic game of basketball with friends for half an hour, then go home to study for an hour before going to bed early?

**4  You have been asked to take part in a fun run three weeks from now. Do you:**

a) Decide that there is no way you could ever run that far, and say "No"?
b) Go running every lunch at school and every evening with an adult, until you pull a muscle in your leg and cannot take part?
c) Go running at school at recess and with an adult once or twice a week, to build up your speed and stamina?

**5  Your friend calls to ask you to go for a bicycle ride. Your mom says it is OK. Do you:**

a) Dash around to your friend's house?
b) Grab your bicycle helmet before you leave?
c) Change your clothes, pack a water bottle, check that your bike is working, and put your helmet on, then go to your friend's house?

## Answers

Mostly **as**: Exercise does not seem very important to you! Try starting with a little exercise each week. You will soon get going!

Mostly **bs**: You are probably exercising for about an hour a day, which is great. But there is more you can do to get even more exercise.

Mostly **cs**: You are a real exercise expert! Congratulations—and keep it up.

# Glossary

**able-bodied** To be healthy and have no illness, injury, or condition that makes it hard to do things that other people do.

**aerobic** Energetic exercise that makes your heart and lungs work harder.

**balanced diet** Eating the right types and amounts of different food.

**community** A place where people live, such as a village or town.

**disabled** To have a condition that makes it hard to do the things that other people do.

**endorphins** Chemicals in the brain that can make you feel happy and relaxed.

**evaporates** Disappears.

**fit** Healthy and strong.

**flexible** When your body can bend easily without breaking.

**flushed** When your face becomes red.

**fuel** A substance that gives us energy and strength.

**joint** Where two bones are connected.

**martial arts** A traditional Japanese or Chinese form of fighting or defending yourself. Karate and kung fu are both martial arts.

**minerals** Important substances found in many foods that are good for your health.

**muscles** Tissues in the body that can tighten and relax so that you can move.

**oxygen** A type of gas found in the air we breathe. We need oxygen to live.

**pedometer** A device used to measure how far you have walked, by counting how many times you lift and put down your feet.

**physical** To do with the body.

**reflective** Can be seen easily, especially when it is dark.

**stamina** The ability to do something for a long time.

**strength** The ability to do something that needs a lot of physical effort.

**sunscreen** A lotion or cream you put on your skin to prevent it from burning in the sun.

**tendons** Strong cords in the body that connect muscle to bone.

**vitamins** Substances found in many foods that are good for your health.

**weights** Heavy objects that people lift for exercise.

**whole food** Food that contains all parts of a grain, such as wheat or oats, with nothing taken away.

# Find out more and Web Sites

**Books**

*Do It Yourself: Keeping Fit* by Carol Ballard (Heinemann Educational Books, 2008)

*Frequently Asked Questions About Exercise Addiction* by Edward Willett (Rosen Publishing Group, 2008)

*The How and Why of Exercise: What Happens to Your Body When You Run* by Simone Payment (Rosen Central, 2009)

**Web Sites**

Due to the changing nature of Internet links, PowerKids Press has developed an online list of Web sites related to the subject of this book. This site is updated regularly. Please use this link to access this list: http://www.powerkidslinks.com/bhfg/exerc/

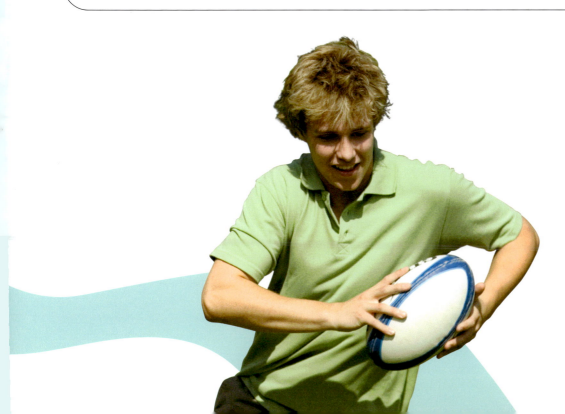

# Index